Between Time and Space

E.S.T.

By Old Nick / Nick Peterson

Contents

ISBN 978-1-7374850-9-4

Published by DiaryUnlimited Imprint: The Edge Press, a division of Global Edge Mnemonics LLC, USA.

Summary

The effects of living on its own for a human or any other members of the animal kingdom either deaf, mute or even blind and the possibility of time-travel.

This is an experiment with time and the mind.

Selected people are forced to live in separate rooms in the dark for a month and they can't see or hear each other. The house is riddled with "night-vision" cameras. Each day the contestants will be undergoing an "auditing" and interview process.

The only way anyone can depart from his living condition to a different time and universe is by cleaning the mind and the soul, a process that can only be obtained by living in the dark.

Characters

X1: Old Nick

X2: John Waterhouse

X3: Mark Joseph

X4: Jenia Emmanuelle

X5: Jonathan Cross

Dr Kelvin: James Hogan

Chapter 1: Exhibit 1. Map of the Universe

Dr Kelvin: This experiment is called E.S.T. There is no escape for the duration of the entire process, no matter the state of the "patient".

Ordinary madness tends to fascinate our society because we both fear it and chase it desperately. Some fight the damn scoundrel and some can't have enough of it. Madness is letting our brain believe that anything could happen. Anything will happen if one allows it. It's only the madness, which is a figment of imagination. The impossible happens. It has not been imagined. Imagination is truer than reality. It is our present tense.

This is an experiment with time and the mind.

The first thing to notice about the Universe is that the solar system is mostly empty space. The planets are very small in comparison to the space between them. To navigate through the planet, we need an evolving map, the "Map of the Universe".

Selected people are forced to live in separate rooms in the dark for a month and they can't see or hear each other. The house is riddled with "night-vision" cameras. Each day the patients will be undergoing an "auditing" and interview process.

The only way anyone can depart from his living condition to a different time and universe is by cleaning the mind and the soul, a process that can only be obtained by living in the dark.

Living in the dark is the most fascinating experience:

-In the dark eating and drinking is slowed down and the whole digestion process works better.

-In the dark we live longer

-In the dark we can control our breathing better

-In the dark sex is orgasmic

-In the dark anything can be cured

-In the dark when the mind is finally free it can travel to a different time and universe

Chapter 2: Exhibit 2:

Venus. Submitting to the authority.

X1: *sleeping*

X3: *sleeping*

X4: *sleeping*

Chapter 3: Exhibit 3.

Saturn. Acknowledging Submission.

X1: *being observed.*

Chapter 4: Exhibit 4. Mercury. Obedience.

Dr. Kelvin: What do you remember? What do you really remember? That is the question. And if we would allow our brain to do just that then we might just get away with living the perfect future!

X3: I thought it would be interesting. This is not exactly what I expected. I don't expect to be I don't know, to have your whole life churned out of you like a therapist.

This is not what I had in mind for a game show. But, I guess, that's the way it is. So, what d'you wanna know?

I want and it might be, it's a funny one. I used to think I knew her really well. But, then, every day she does something, says something, and just think there's a lot I don't know. So, she's around.

That's all you get, you know, you see the outside, it's fun doing things, you go places, everything's great. But the inside's always a bit of a mystery.

That's not really the way it manifested. It was... different. There's been people in the past where that's all it was. You meet them, fuck 'em, chuck 'em, that's it. But, her...That's what Jane, that's who she is.

Chapter 5: Exhibit 5. Uranus. Transcending.

X1: *being observed.*

Chapter 6: Exhibit 6. Titan. Complete Annihilation.

X3: I did have some fun. How to understand: the whole world is there watching everything? But this is not the end of the world. To answer this? I did it! When you're 10 years' s you stick something up your veins, snort something up your nose and you do it because your parents told you not to because you might die. Then you get older and you try things with friends and you don't die and you do it again and again and you get older and you get bored and you stop.

Chapter 7: Exhibit 7. Mars. Transmitting.

X1: *being observed*

Chapter 8: Exhibit 8.

Neptune. Remembering, absorbing the thought.

X3: You ask quite obtrusive questions, don't you? But, to answer I did have them but not as a rule. How can you not? The person is your whole world, everything to you, there's something and at the time, it's not like the end of the world, you know, when you're 10 years old sticking something in your veins, snorting something up your nose seems like the worst thing in the world, you know, your parents have told you not to because you might die.   Then, when you get older, you try thing sin clubs, you try things with friends, and you don't die. So, you do it again, and again, and again. And then when you get older you get bored and start... but I'm not there yet. I don't know.

Drugs are funny. You know when you see a homeless person, drinking, asking for money, you walk past them and say tut, tut, tut, if I only give them money, they're going to spend it on drink. Go and buy some food.

They don't want fucking food. You know, a sandwich doesn't make you forget who you are. You know. They drink because

they don't want to be fucking lying on the floor. If you're pissed out of your face, you could be anywhere.

I mean, I'm not homeless but I've had plenty of times where I don't want to be where I am right now and drugs are just a way there.

So, I've been to other places. I've... flown to other dimensions [sighs] and honestly, sometimes I mean, I've been in that negative dimension on my own with Jane and with anyone. Sometimes I don't want to come back. And after a while... kind of just completely live there. We belong there. And that's dangerous.

Turn to, not really turn to anyone. There are people around, you know, I know people who have friends. So, I see people here and there but, to be frank, I don't mind being on my own. I can deal with it. When you're on your own there's no-one to piss you off. You can do what you want. Say what you want. No-one's going to bitch at you. Live where you want; eat what you want; drink what you want.   And no-one says a word, if they're not there.

Chapter 9: Exhibit 9. The Moon. Thoughts gathering: seeking to express and communicate.

X1: *being observed*

Chapter 10: Exhibit 10. Earth. Defiance.

X5: My name is Jonathan. I live here. Sometimes. No. I've never thought about committing suicide or anything like that. I've only taken drugs twice or three times in my life. Yes, I have sex. If I can I have sex with someone. Yes. Yes. I have. Oh, London is full of crap. You come home, blow your nose, it's...   If I can't sleep and I'm bored I will try to have sex. I do masturbate sometimes. Hmm. Umm, truthfully, I would masturbate about twice or three times a month.   No, it's not unhealthy to masturbate at all. I'm 23.

Chapter 11: Exhibit 11.   Jupiter. Abnegation.

X1: *being observed*

Chapter 12: Exhibit 12. IO Resilience.

X3: Yeah. Really fine, don't worry. I can see spaces.

She's everywhere. She's in my head. You know when you think about someone so much that they're always near you, she could be anywhere. Some people you know and you don't even have to see them for very long, you might see them for 10 minutes every six months, as long as you know where they are, that's enough. I don't know. She, um, she's always right here. Even though I hardly ever know where she is.

Under water. Everything is just the same. You know, I thought I could escape the world, go somewhere different, be in another world. But, when it comes down to it, they're all the same.

Things killing each other. Things fucking each other. All day long. It gets hot, it gets cold, it's just the same. I didn't escape anywhere. Sometimes you can't… you feel like you can't breathe sometimes free as a bird.

All these worlds are exactly the same. Just different. Saw things. Well, I think I saw things, you never really know. I saw people I interacted in a world that, ah, I never even knew was there. In ways I didn't even know I could. And just I felt like I couldn't live in this place anymore. So, I went somewhere else.

Either it was too hot, I couldn't, I couldn't manage. Everything was too new, too shit, I couldn't... but, then, you get used to it. And it becomes normal. Even the shit becomes normal. You get used to the shit, and believe me there's a fuck load of shit everywhere just like here.

You know, here, London, wherever, shit all over the place, garbage, rubbish on the floor, pollution, bullshit. In the water, same thing; bodies floating all over the place. Fishes fucking cacking all over the place. Seaweed all over the place covering everything like garbage. It's just the same. And when you can breathe, when it's not too stifling, then you start to think normal things again, well, I say normal, I keep thinking about killing is generally regarded as normal by many people except me.

I think most people think about killing. But never seriously. It's never an actual choice or a topic of conversation. You know. Everyone says 'oh yeah, I'd kill Hitler kill it. But, would they? No. But, when I think about it, I think about it like it's an art. Now, I'm no serial killer. But there is a certain beauty in killing. A purity. I never thought of myself as someone who had a conscience like that but to see yourself in another way is a bit of a mind fuck because sometimes, I didn't even know if I was right. You know, usually, it's you versus a fucked-up version of you and you're right, he's wrong. And it's until you sort out that problem that he goes away. But, this time, I didn't know if I was right because some of the things he said, they just made so much sense.   But, sometimes, I wish he was always here. Sometimes I wish he was in the fucking driving seat up here because, sometimes, I don't know what I'm doing and I feel that he does. More than me. I don't know; I don't really see him as a guardian angel. More some mother-fucker that has access to my head and sometimes chooses to work the controls

Chapter 13: Exhibit 13. Europa. Acceptance, transmitting...

X1: *being observed*

Chapter 14: Exhibit 14. Triton. Transmission.

X4: I'm tired of this game and I want to sleep, okay?
Do you understand?

Chapter 15: Exhibit 15. Cheron. Space / time travel.

X1: *being observed*

Chapter 16: Exhibit 16. Callisto. Controlled.

X2: X. You can call me X. if you want. Some people do. Well, I've been trying to forget what happened and the mad guy, he's quite nice and, um, I guess you know. I've just been trying to find things to do here and find my way. I don't know. She's weird. When you do something, how big, how it can change you, how you can become a totally different person, you know. Maybe in the past but I've changed. People change, you know. I'm sure you do. I used to smoke, I used to drink. I guess thinking I killed someone was good for me in some ways, you know. I stopped drinking, stopped smoking; people should kill more often. I used to do drugs and drink and everything and it just changed me. It changed me totally. No. Not really. Why should I be scared? What do you want from me?   I think I've told you all I have to tell you now. What else is there to say? Nothing.

Do I miss her?

Yes. I miss her. Even when I'm with her because I know she's not always with me.

You know when sometimes you're with someone but you can see in their eyes, they're somewhere else

That's what I see with Jane a lot.

Chapter 17: Exhibit 17. Pluto. Away.

X1: *being observed*

Chapter 18: Exhibit 18. Sun. Complete annihilation.

X4: I want happiness, a successful career and love. Well, I've changed. If it's the right person, I'm into sex.

All I know is, is, things did not end well. Well, when someone dies it's not going to end well.   I don't know what she was doing with him or what he was doing with someone else. But, from experience, Jane is not someone you want to fuck with in that way.

She's someone you want to fuck with but not fuck with, if you get what I mean. Well, anyway, he was fucking with someone else. I guess she just took care of the situation. If you know what I mean.

For me? Why have you put me in this room? Why am I hear anyway? Say something. What do you want from me? What do you want? Why am I here? What am I doing here? What do you want? I don't understand. I want to get out of here; I don't like it anymore, okay? I don't like it here anymore. I want you to let me go. I know I signed up to be in this game show but I don't want to be in it anymore, okay, I don't... I don't want to be in it anymore, do you understand?

Just let me out of here. Please, I don't want to be in this show anymore. I don't like it. I don't like being in this show anymore, just… please let me out. I want to be out of this show. I don't't' like it anymore.

X2: I'm Fine. Perfect. How do I know Jane? Yes, we are. I don't know. Maybe in London. Of course, I like her. No, she's not my girlfriend. She used to be my wife. No X2, what X2? I don't know any X2. Of course, I am. No, I don't have a surname.

What is this noise? … My first and only name I already told you. What do you mean? Where are you? I know where I'm. I don't remember. I had an accident I fell into a coma. What is that noise? I don't remember I don't remember I don't remember I don't remember I don't remember I don't remember… Have we finished now? I don't remember. What question is that? Of course, I have a mother! Pause What's the point? I have a father!

I don't remember. I don't remember. Can we stop now? Can we stop now? I'm sorry…

I'm not feeling well. Are you listening to me or what? I'm not well.

Fuck with X2, I don't know any X2 Maybe I do know a X2 I don't remember I don't remember; I don't remember.

What's that noise?

A long time, quite a long time ago.

I'm sleepy, I want to sleep. I want to rest. Would you let me get out now? I want to get out now!

Fuck with Jane. You can call her if you want. Let me get out now, please, I want to get out. Let me get out.

Can you hear me, doctor? I want to get out! Pause I'm cold I want to sleep; I want to sleep...

Delirious. Barely audible. I'm on the sofa now. I'm on the sofa now. I'm on the sofa now. I'm on the sofa now.

I want to get out now, I want to get out now. Now, now, now!

His voice is slowly fading away. The Unit of measurement displayed on the screen is dangerously high. The red color is going out of control.

Now, now! Yes. I had an accident. A car. A car hit me. A car hit me. I went to hospital. Yes, a coma. A kind of coma.

X2 is about to shout and points the finger at Kelvin and is still lying on the couch unable to move; completely annihilated

Fuck you. No more... I want to get out!

The Unit of measurement explodes on the screen.

X2 is falling gently asleep and whispering.

Y-a, Y-b, Y-c, Y-d, Y-e, Y-f, Y-g, Y-h, Y-I, Y-j, Y-k, Y-l, Y-m, Y-n, Y-o, Y-p, Y-q, Y-r, Y-s, Y-t, Y-u, Y-v, Y-w, Y-x, Y-Y, Y-z.

Chapter 19: Exhibit 19. Pallas.

Navigating between planets.

X1: *being observed.*

Chapter 20: Exhibit 20.

Beyond the Milky Way. Free.

X3: *Escape from his room and find his way to X4.*

Footage of X1, then the Sun.

Exhibit 21. Epilogue.

Dr. Kelvin: What do you remember? What do you really remember? That is the question. And if we would allow our brain to do just that then we might just get away with living the perfect future!

Unfortunately, the solar system has been found to be more complicated than this would suggest: there are several moons larger than Pluto and two larger than Mercury; there are many small moons that are probably started out as asteroids and were only later captured by a planet; Comets sometimes fizzle out and become indistinguishable from asteroids; Celestial bodies can become quickly irrational, illogical and finally explode. When they do, we can then witness the birth of a black hole. All the black holes merge with one another and they first intoxicate the rest of the universe then eat up every other celestial body in existence. One would then understand the chief importance of keeping each body under tight control.

Chapter 22: End Credits

Characters

X1: Old Nick

X2: John Waterhouse

X3: Mark Joseph

X4: Jenia Emmanuelle

X5: Jonathan Cross

Dr Kelvin: James Hogan

www.ingramcontent.com/pod-product-compliance
Lightning Source LLC
Chambersburg PA
CBHW070259290326
41930CB00041B/2651